Amelia Takes on Cancer

By Amelia Zai

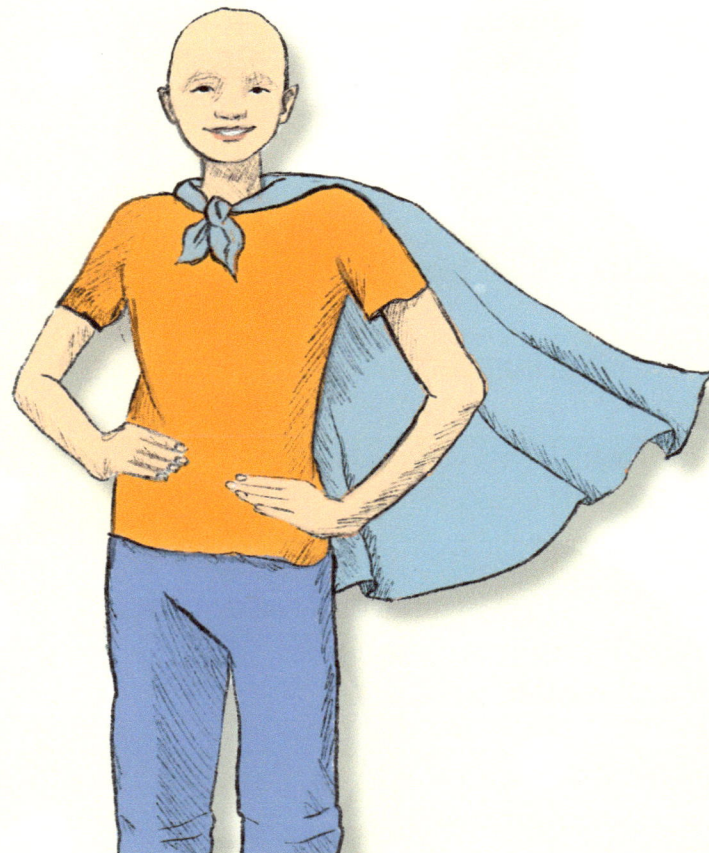

An Interactive Journal for _____

Amelia Takes on Cancer, published August, 2023

Editorial and proofreading services: Katie Barger; Kent Sorsky
Interior layout and cover design: Howard Johnson
Interior and cover artwork creation: Olivia Bosson
Photo Credits: Photos owned by Amelia Zai

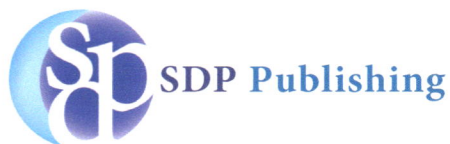

Published by SDP Publishing, an imprint of SDP Publishing Solutions, LLC.

To obtain permission(s) to use material from this work, please submit an email request with subject line:
SDP Publishing Permissions Department.
Email: info@SDPPublishing.com.

ISBN-13 (print): 979-8-9878348-8-6
ISBN-13 (ebook): 979-8-9878348-9-3

To my parents, and the staff and patients at the Jimmy Fund Clinic.

A Word from Amelia

🌼

This book shares my cancer journey and what I learned from it. Even though my story may not be the exact same as yours, I hope it will help you get a sense of what chemotherapy is like. Even though chemotherapy sounds scary, you are not alone in this journey; you have the support of all those around you. Remember that you are strong and that everyone, including me, believes in you!

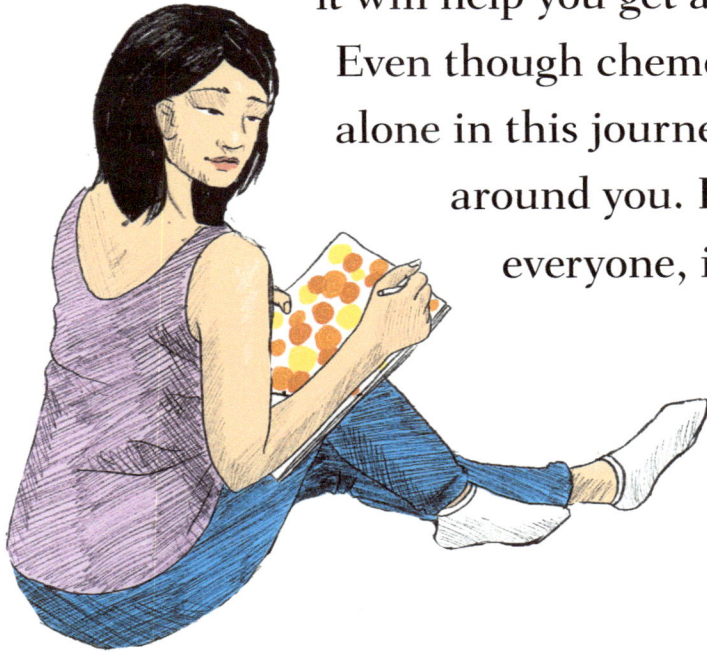

Amelia ♡

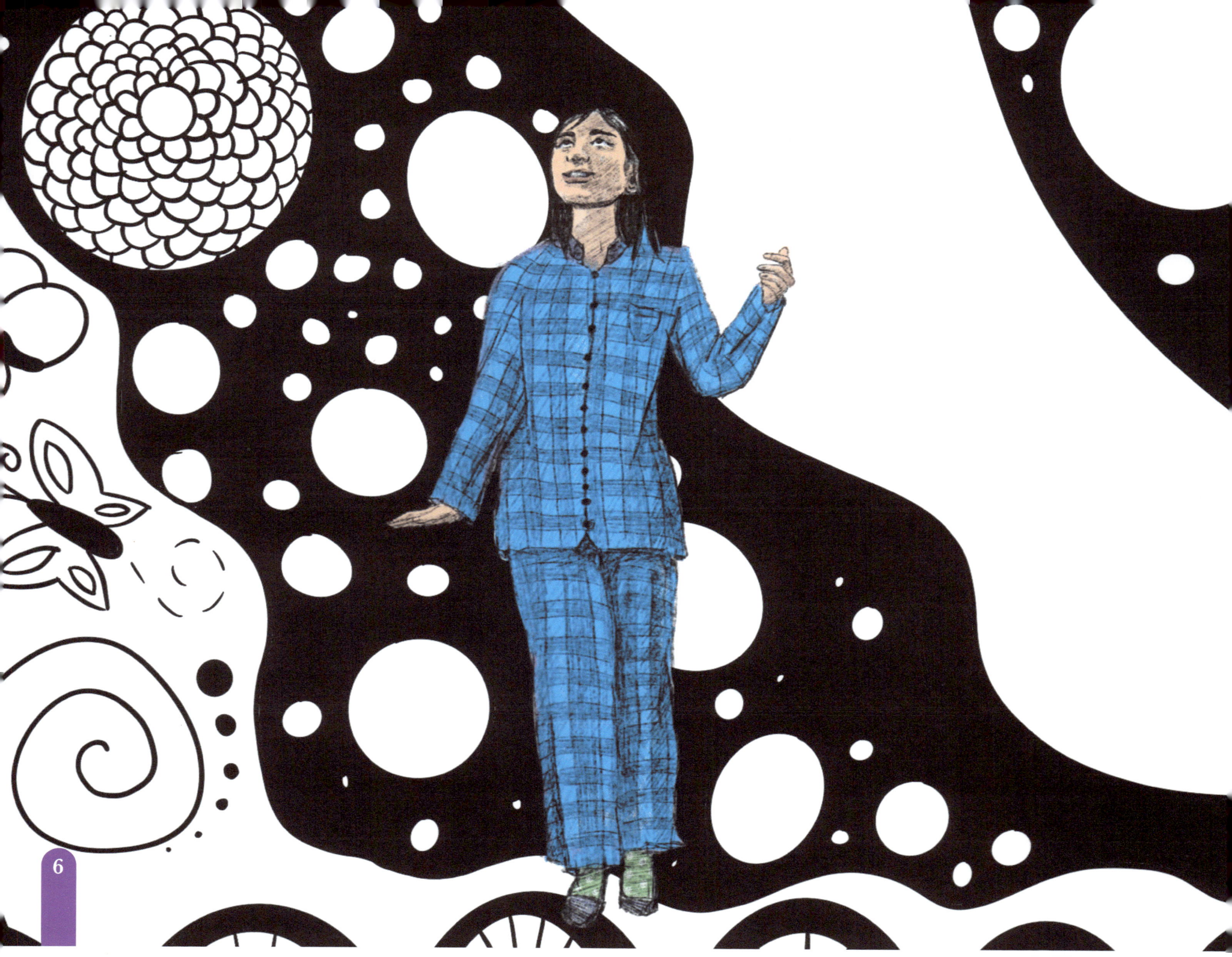

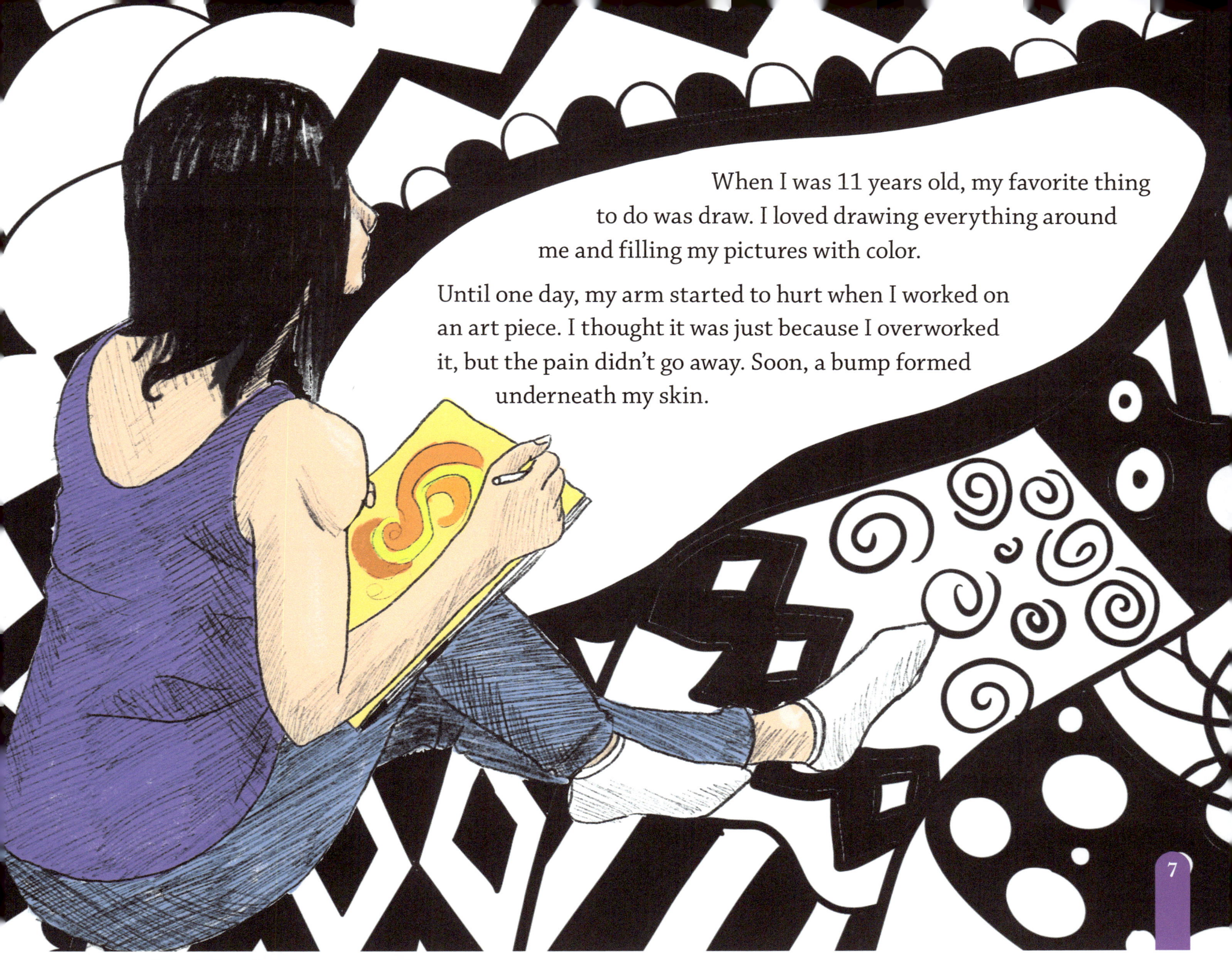

When I was 11 years old, my favorite thing to do was draw. I loved drawing everything around me and filling my pictures with color.

Until one day, my arm started to hurt when I worked on an art piece. I thought it was just because I overworked it, but the pain didn't go away. Soon, a bump formed underneath my skin.

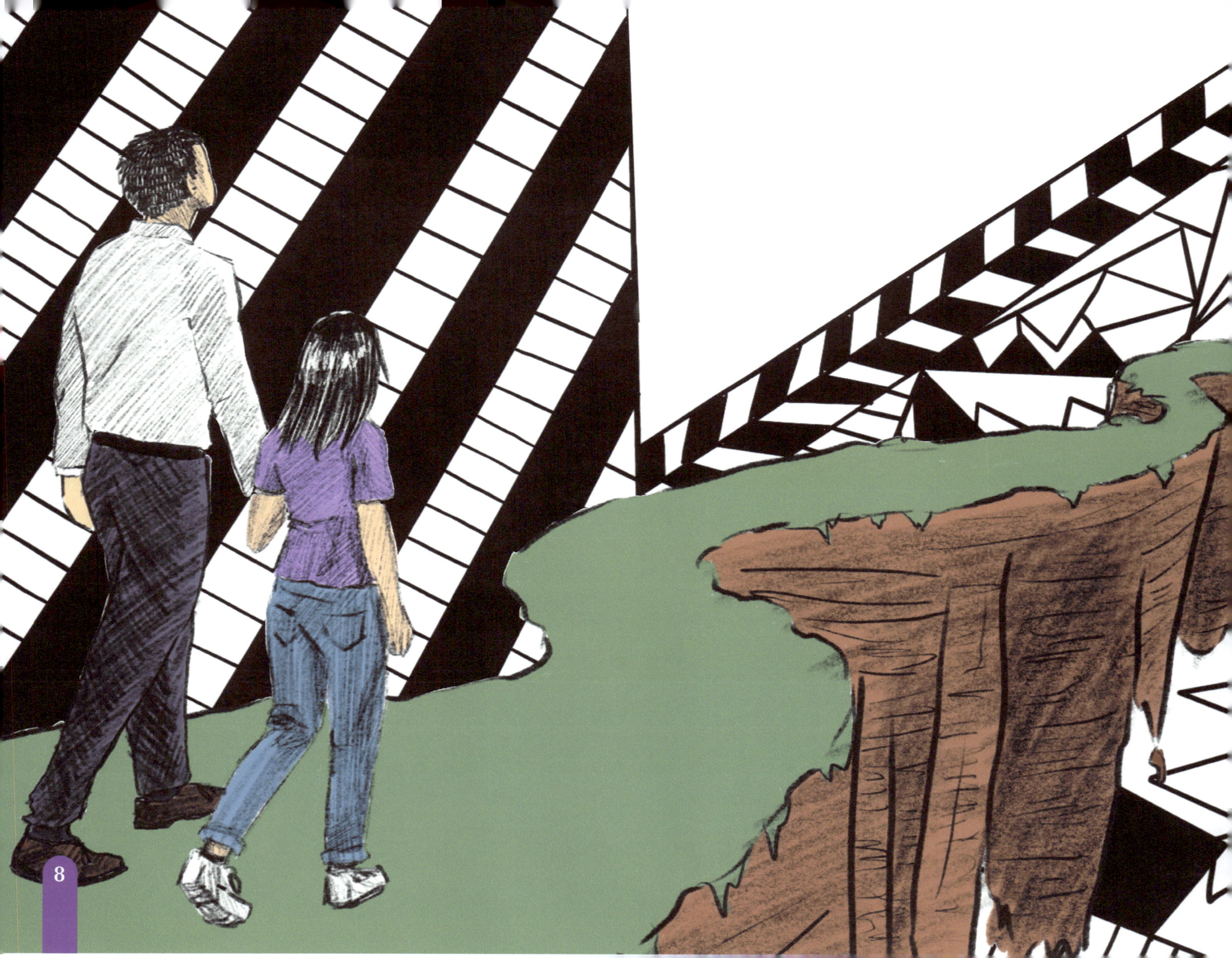

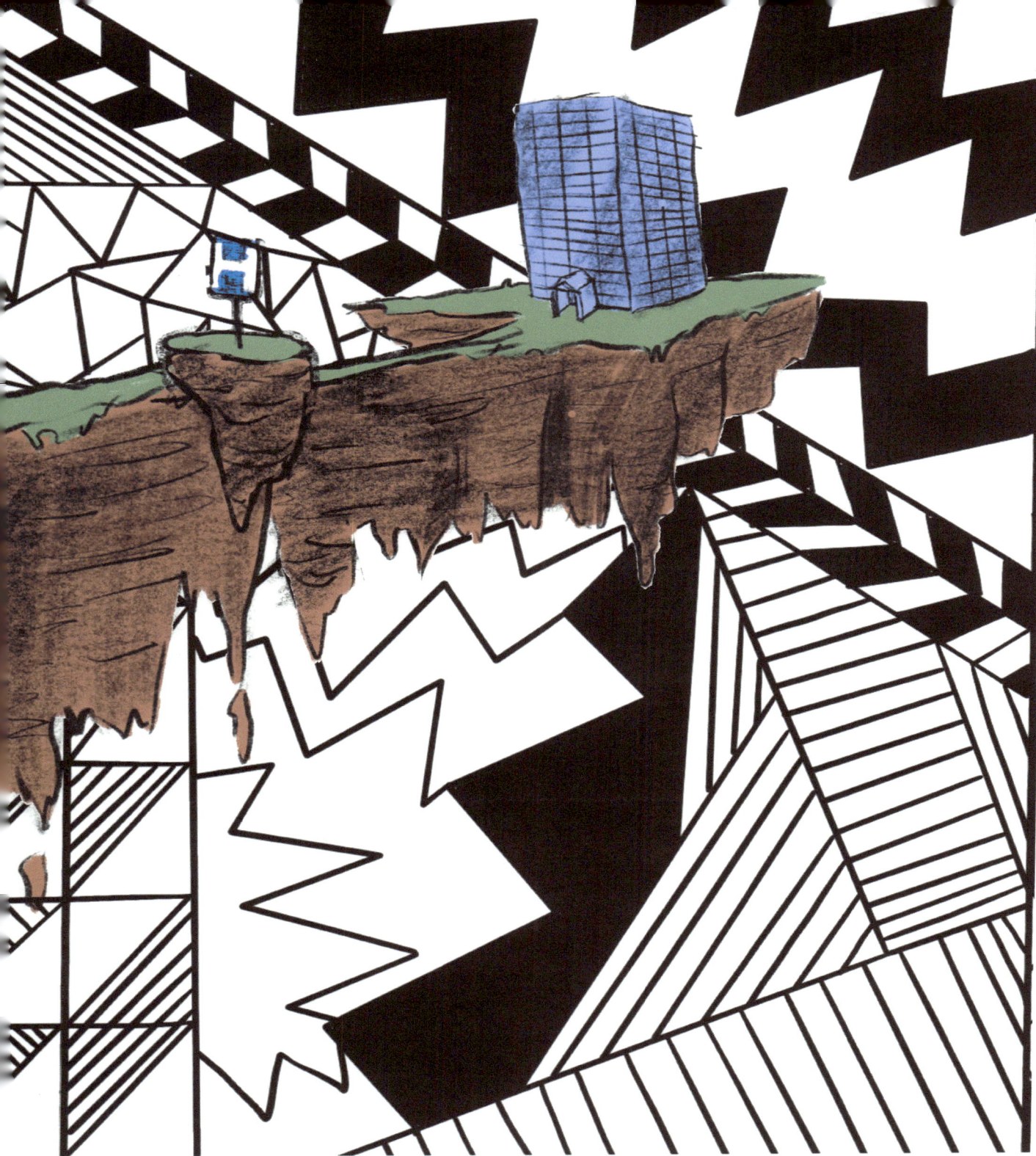

So my dad took me to
see the doctor.

After a few tests, my doctors told me that I had cancer. This is when the cells in your body divide uncontrollably. My doctors told me to come back the following week to create a plan to help me get better.

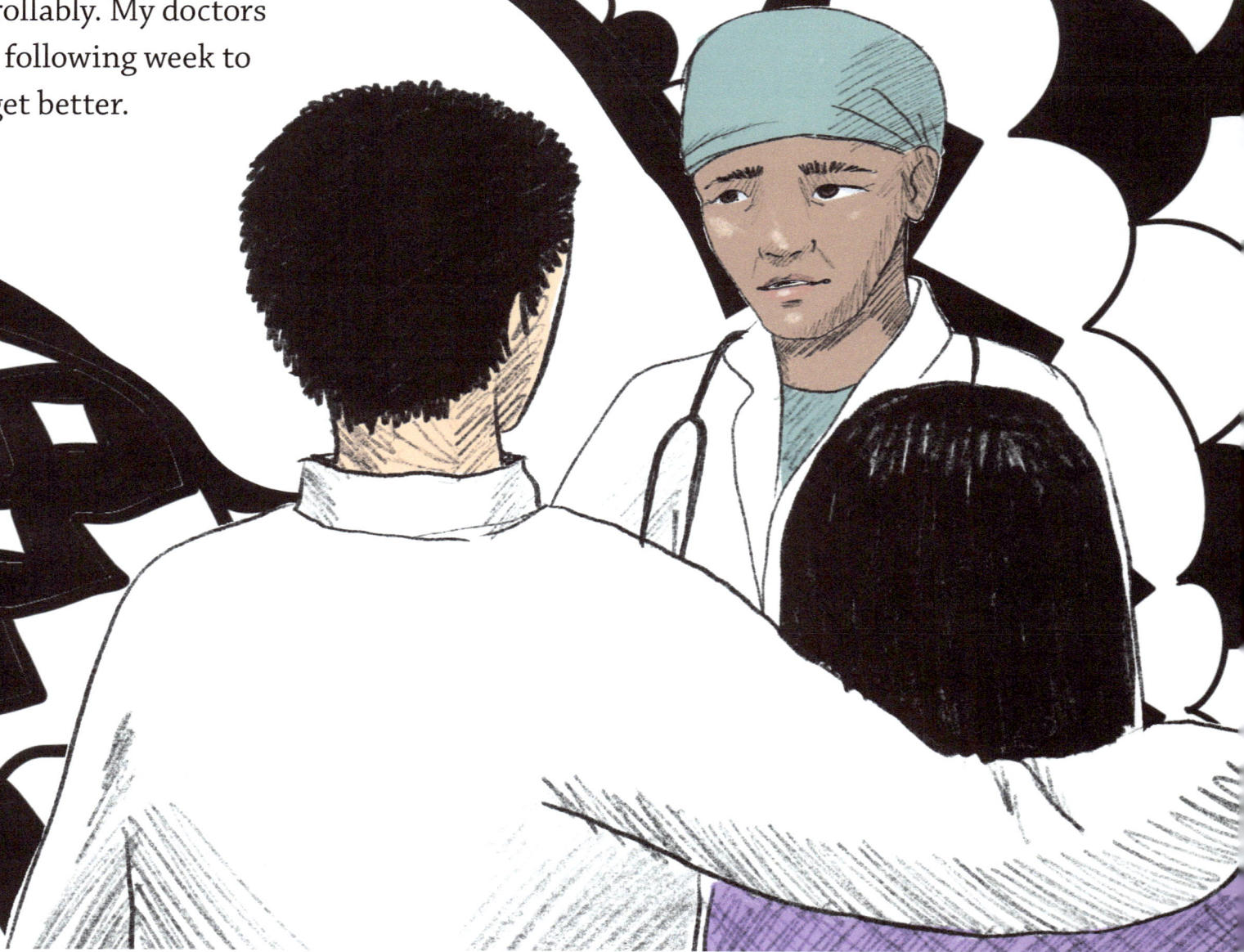

How old were you when you found out you had cancer?

_____

_____

_____

How did you feel?

_____

_____

_____

Were you scared? Confused?

_____

_____

_____

At first, I wasn't worried about what the doctor said. I thought it would be like I had a cold—I'd be better in a week and back to my normal self.

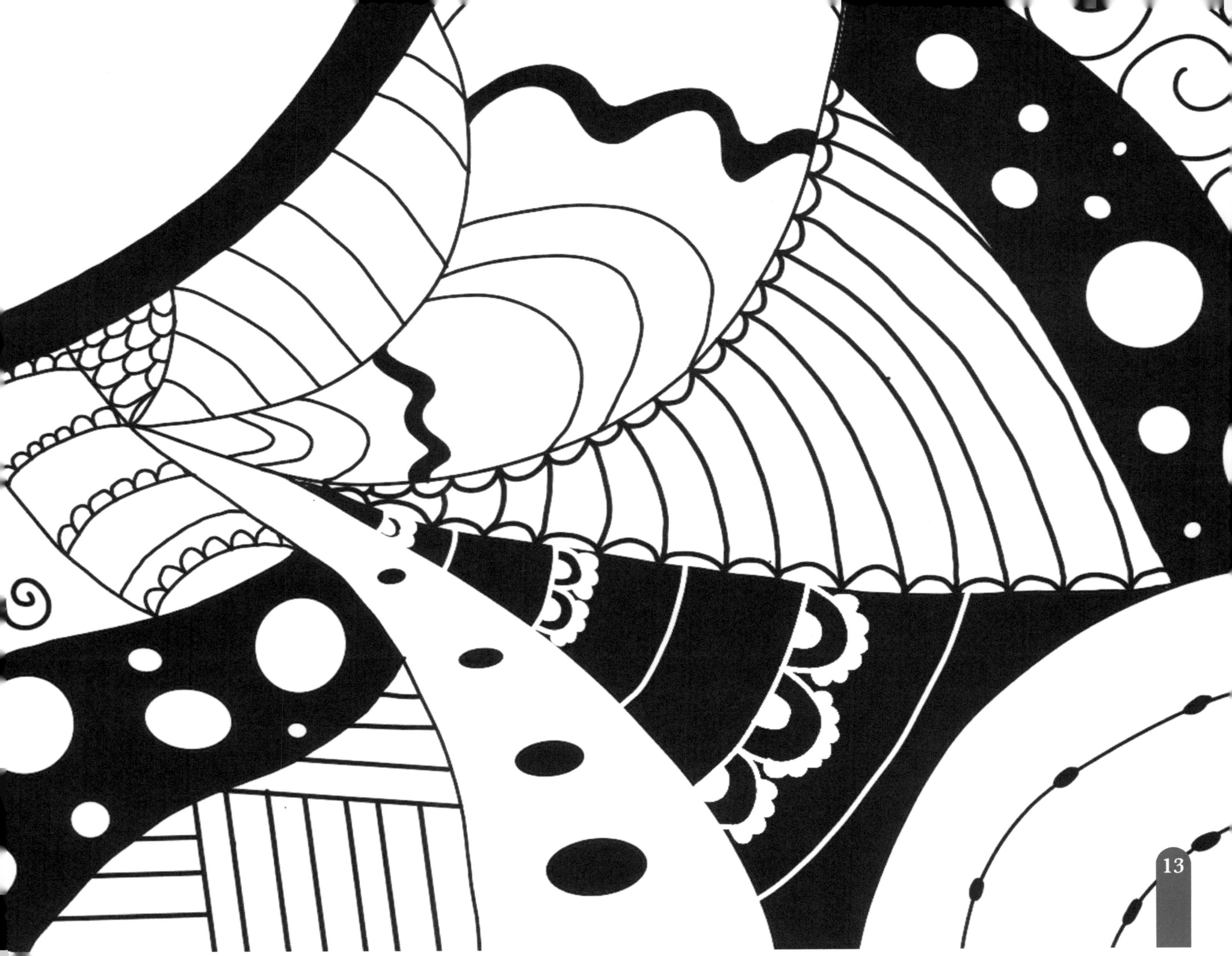

Because I thought I would be better
soon, I decided not to tell anyone about
what happened. I was scared that
people would ask me scary
questions like ...

"Is it contagious?"

"How long will you be sick?"

Or maybe they wouldn't say

anything at all.

Did you tell anyone about your cancer?

_____

_____

_____

Did sharing make you feel better?

_____

_____

_____

_____

_____

_____

_____

When I walked into the clinic the next week for that appointment, I saw kids in the infusion room—a space where kids get cancer medicine called chemotherapy. They all looked scared, yet the room still had a welcoming and positive energy. The doctors told me my best course of action was to get chemotherapy, which meant that soon, I'd be one of those kids in the infusion room. I wasn't excited about that.

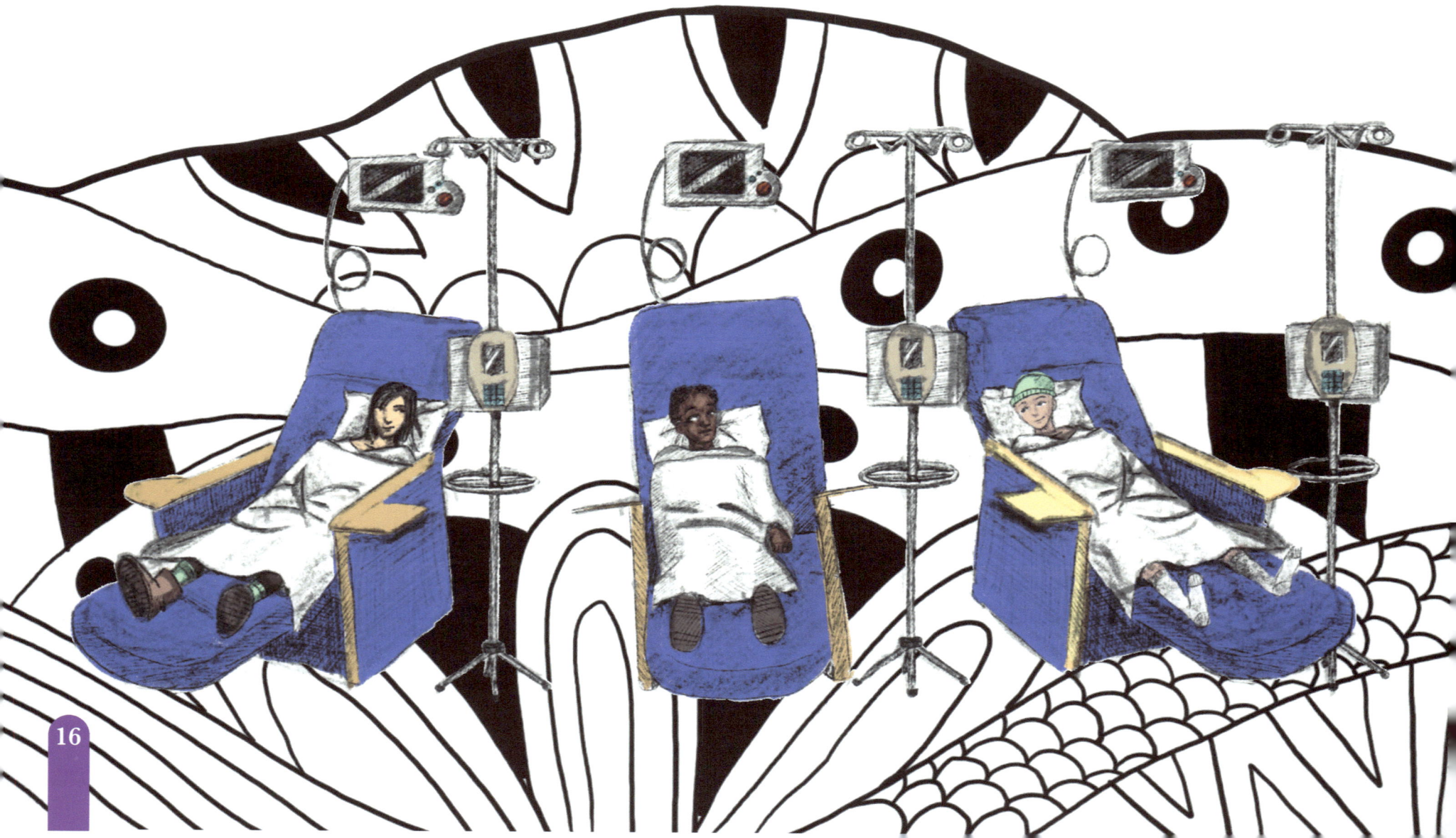

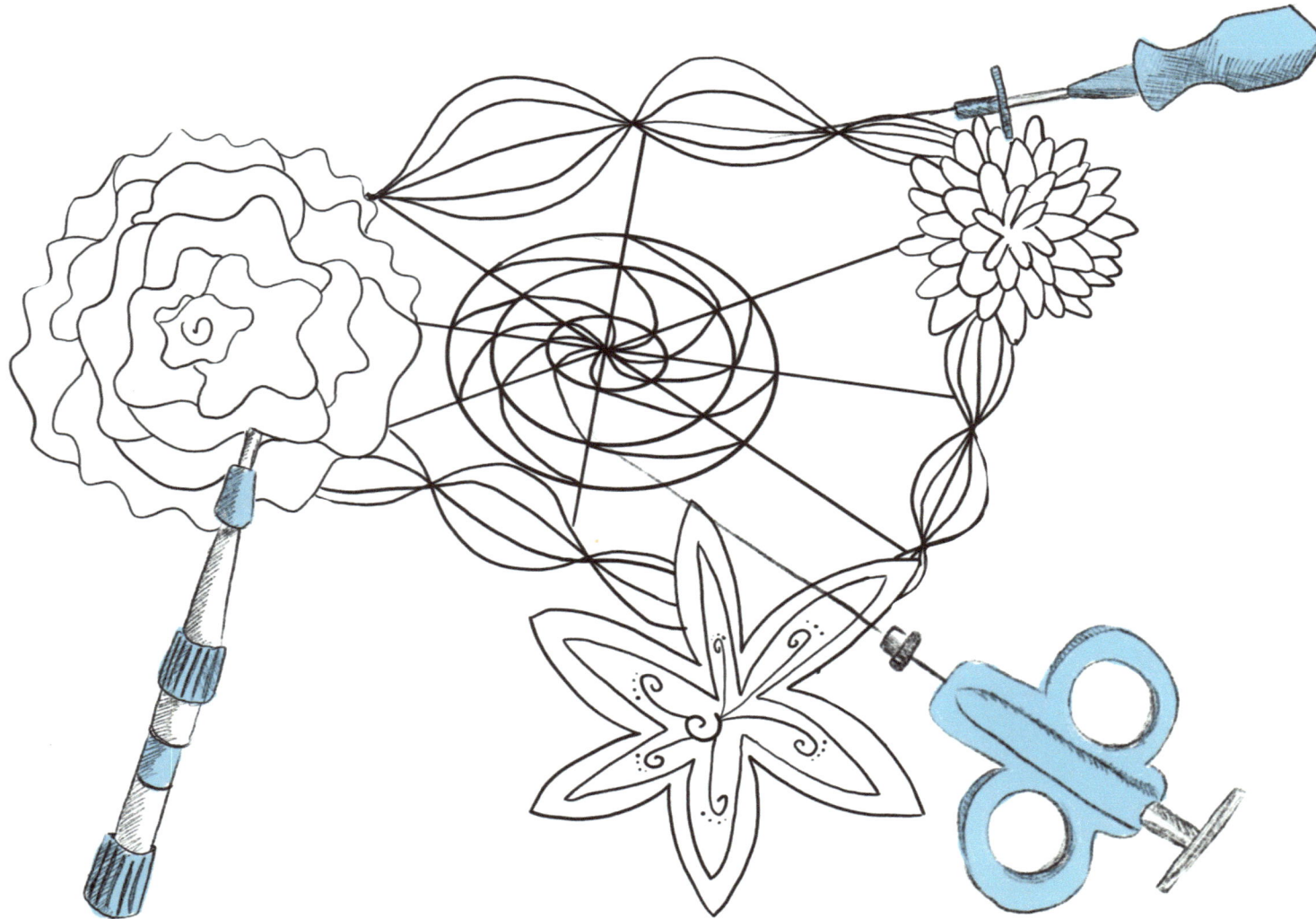

The doctors also recommended that I get a biopsy, which is when doctors take a small piece of tissue from the part of the body where the cancer is located. This sample allowed doctors to figure out what kind of cancer I had. This was the moment I realized it was probably going to take a long time for me to get better. I was terrified.

I was super nervous the morning of my biopsy.
Would it hurt?
Would I be awake during the procedure?

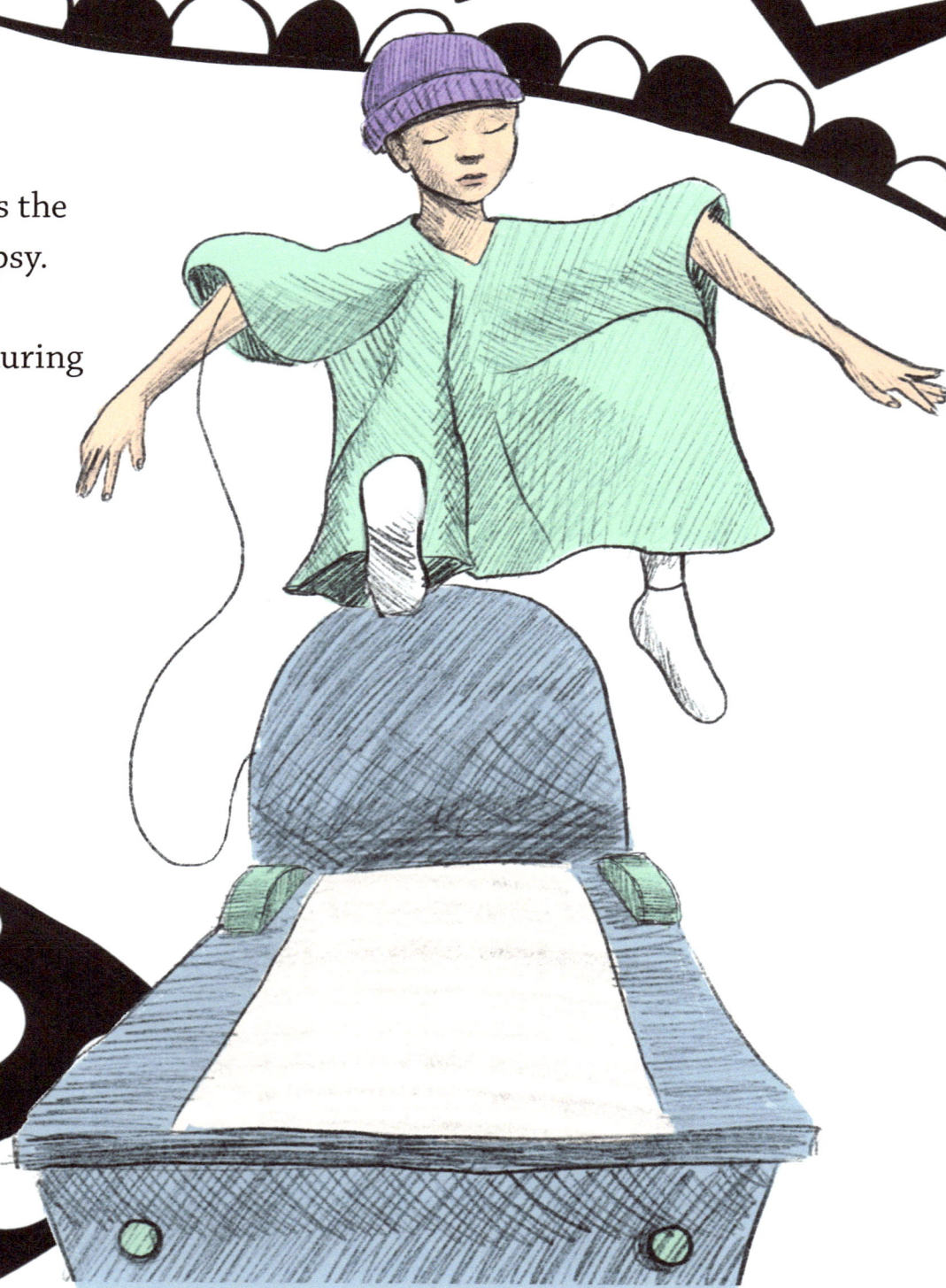

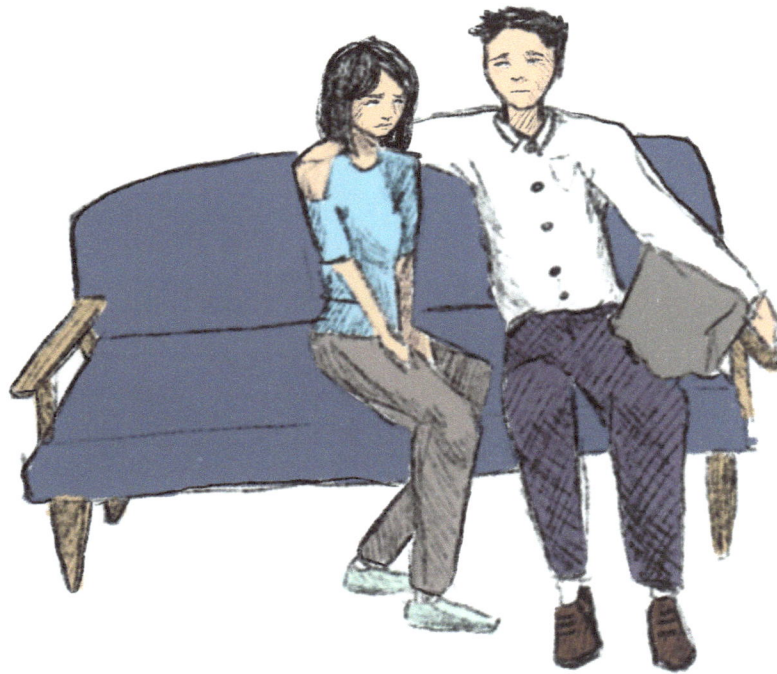

The doctors told me that it wouldn't hurt! They would give me anesthesia, a gas that makes me fall asleep so I wouldn't feel anything.

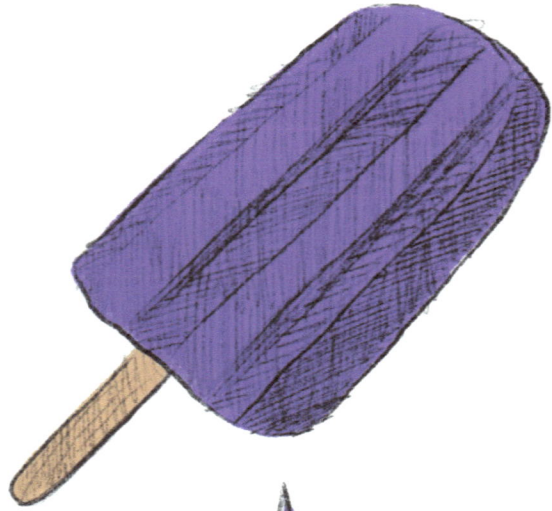

Before I knew it, the procedure was all done, and I was rewarded with a grape popsicle for my bravery.

A few days later, I went back to the hospital to get my biopsy results. A knot wound tighter in my stomach as my parents and I waited to talk to the doctor.

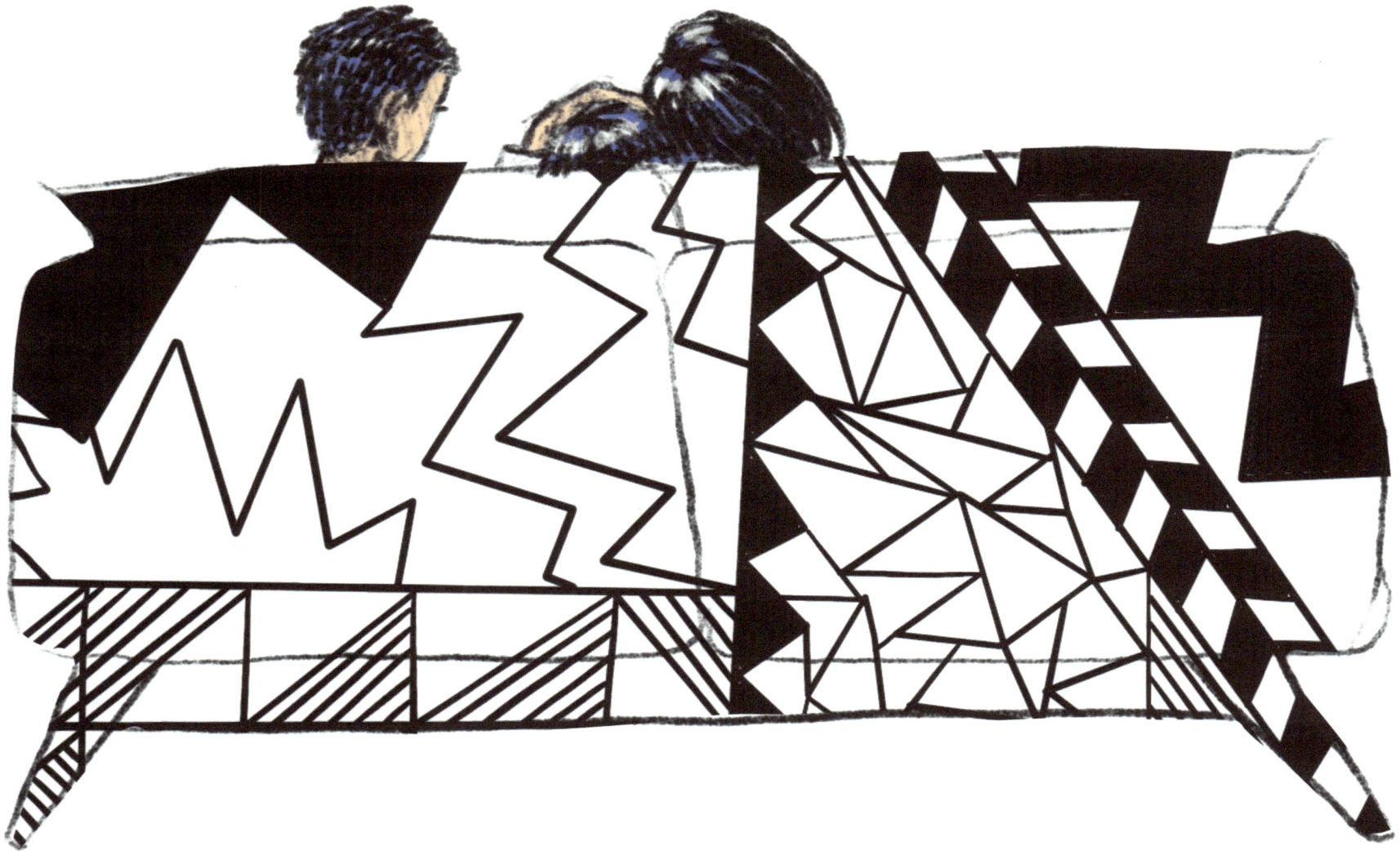

My doctors told me that I had Ewing sarcoma, which usually grows in the bones.

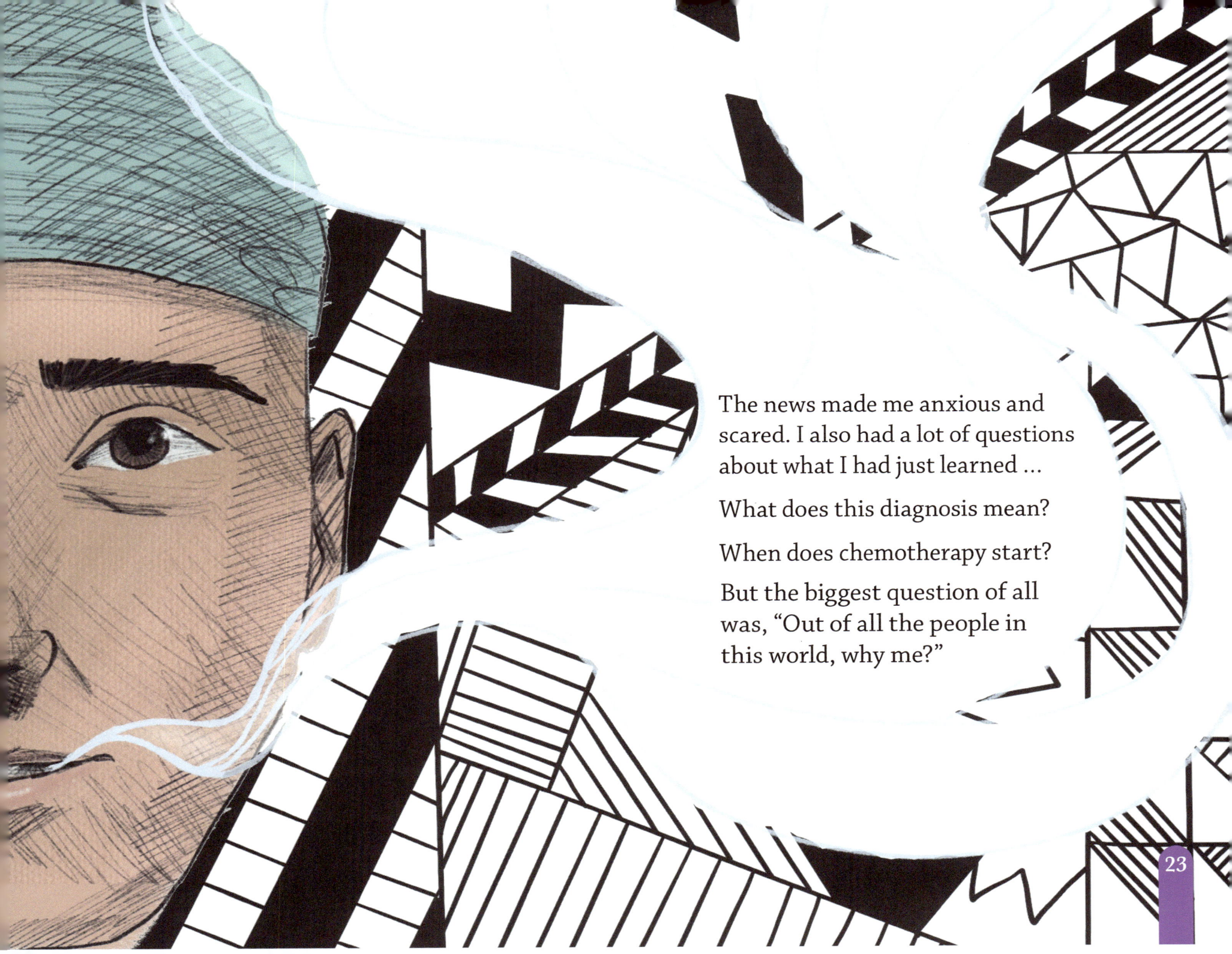

The news made me anxious and scared. I also had a lot of questions about what I had just learned ...

What does this diagnosis mean?

When does chemotherapy start?

But the biggest question of all was, "Out of all the people in this world, why me?"

I started chemotherapy the following week.
Walking into the infusion room wasn't as scary as
I thought it would be. While cleaning my line, a
nurse told me about the snack room.

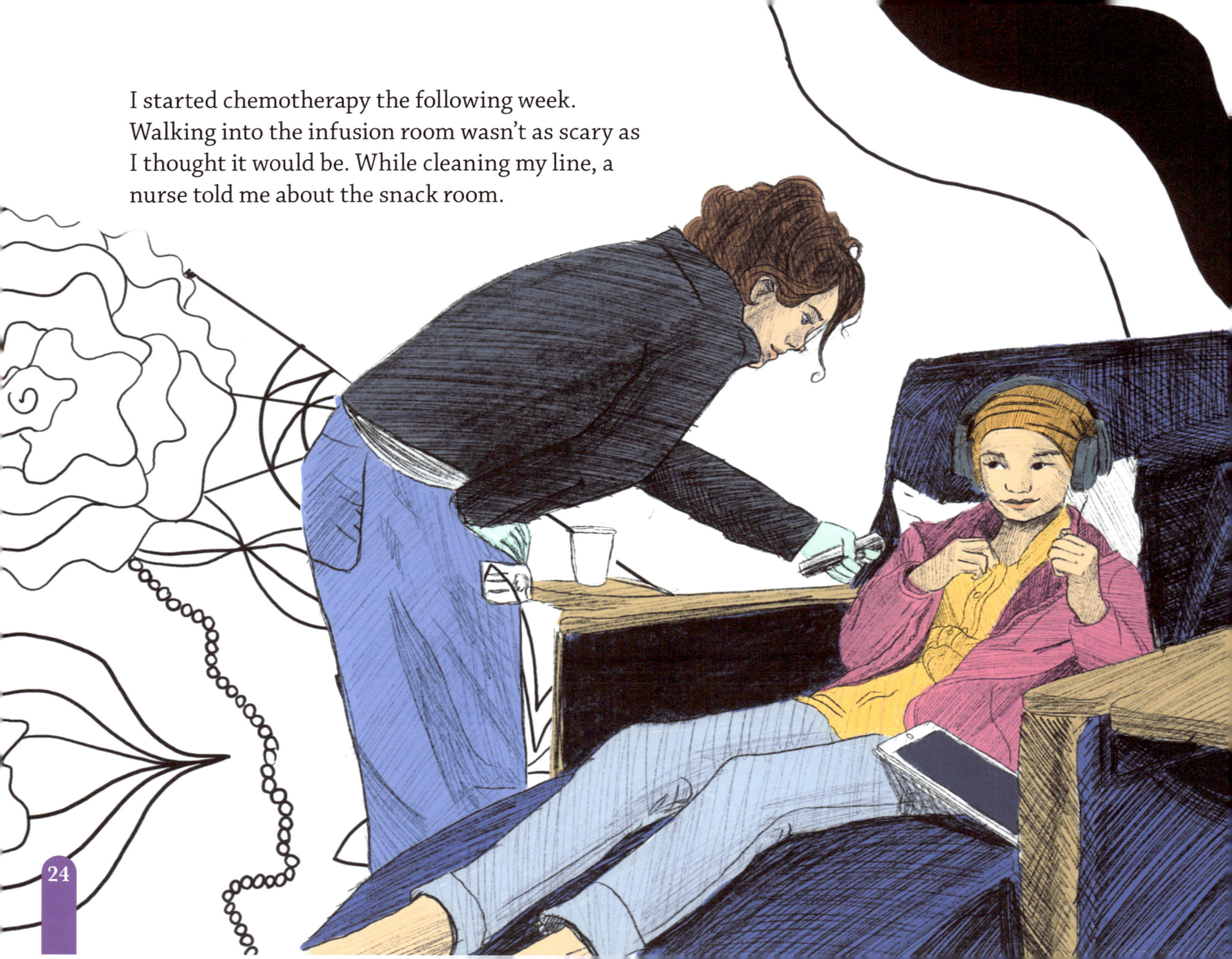

How did you feel walking into the infusion clinic?

_____

_____

_____

_____

What kind of activities does your clinic provide?

_____

_____

_____

_____

_____

_____

I was thrilled to learn that there was a snack bar with some of my favorite snacks and drinks, like cereal and ginger ale!

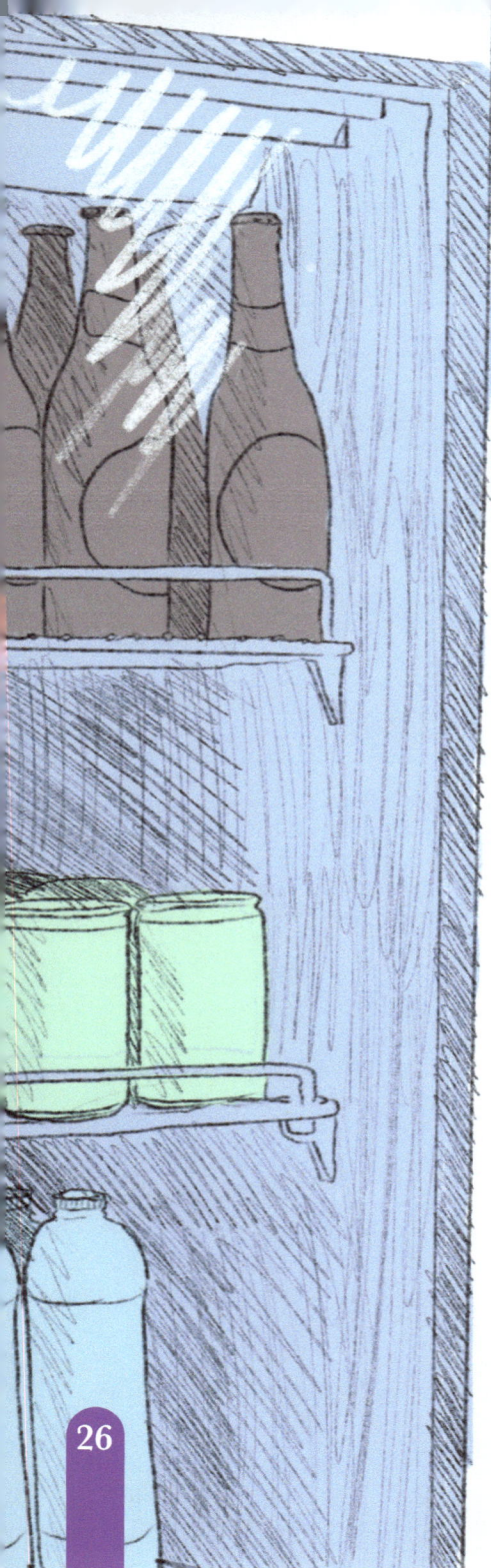

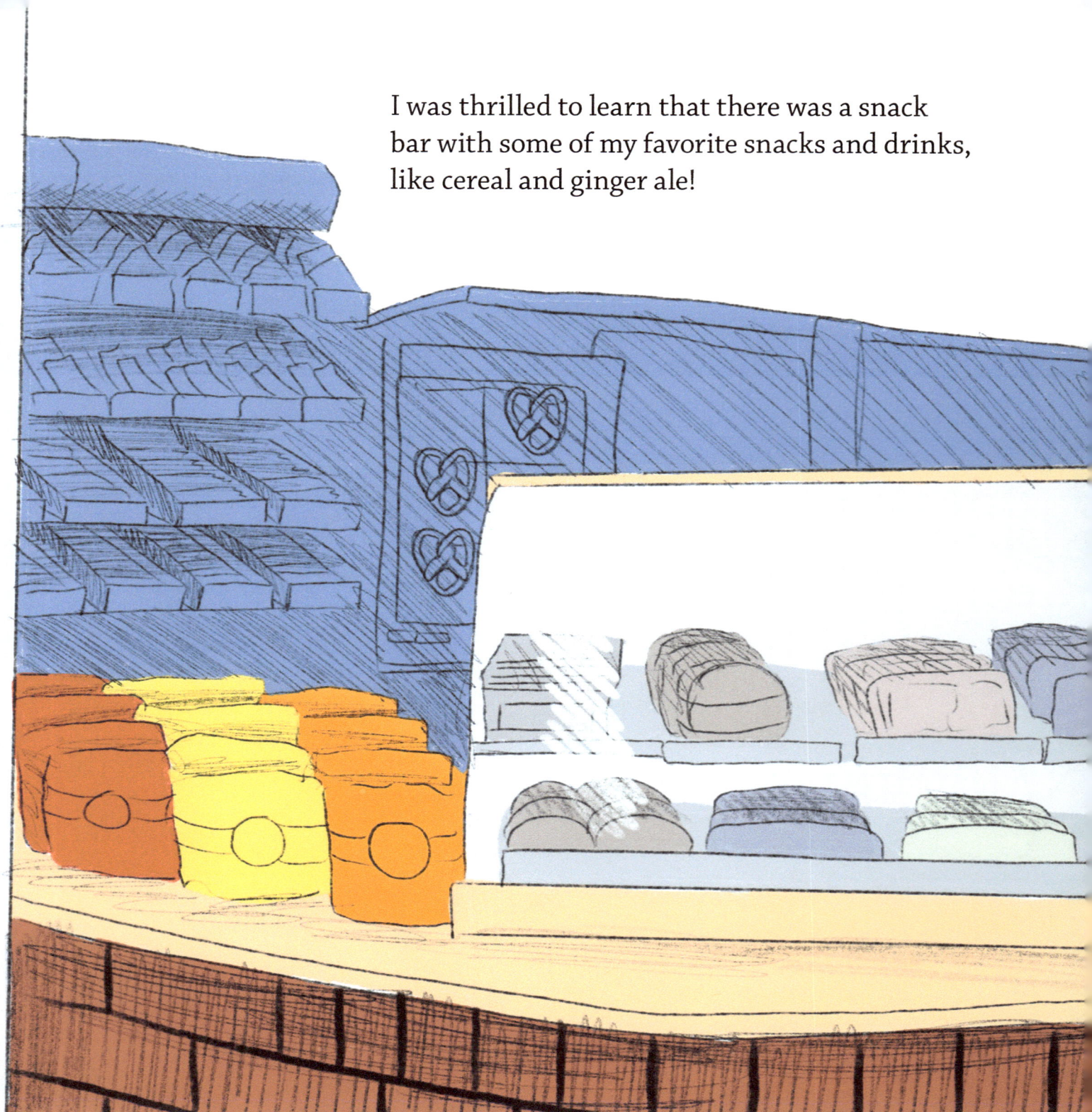

What are your favorite snacks?

_____

_____

You could draw pictures of them here, just like I did!

There was also an activity room for crafts and making new friends.

I had no trouble walking into the snack room and acting like I owned the place, but something about the activity room scared me. It was an unfamiliar space. One day, I built up enough courage to walk in …

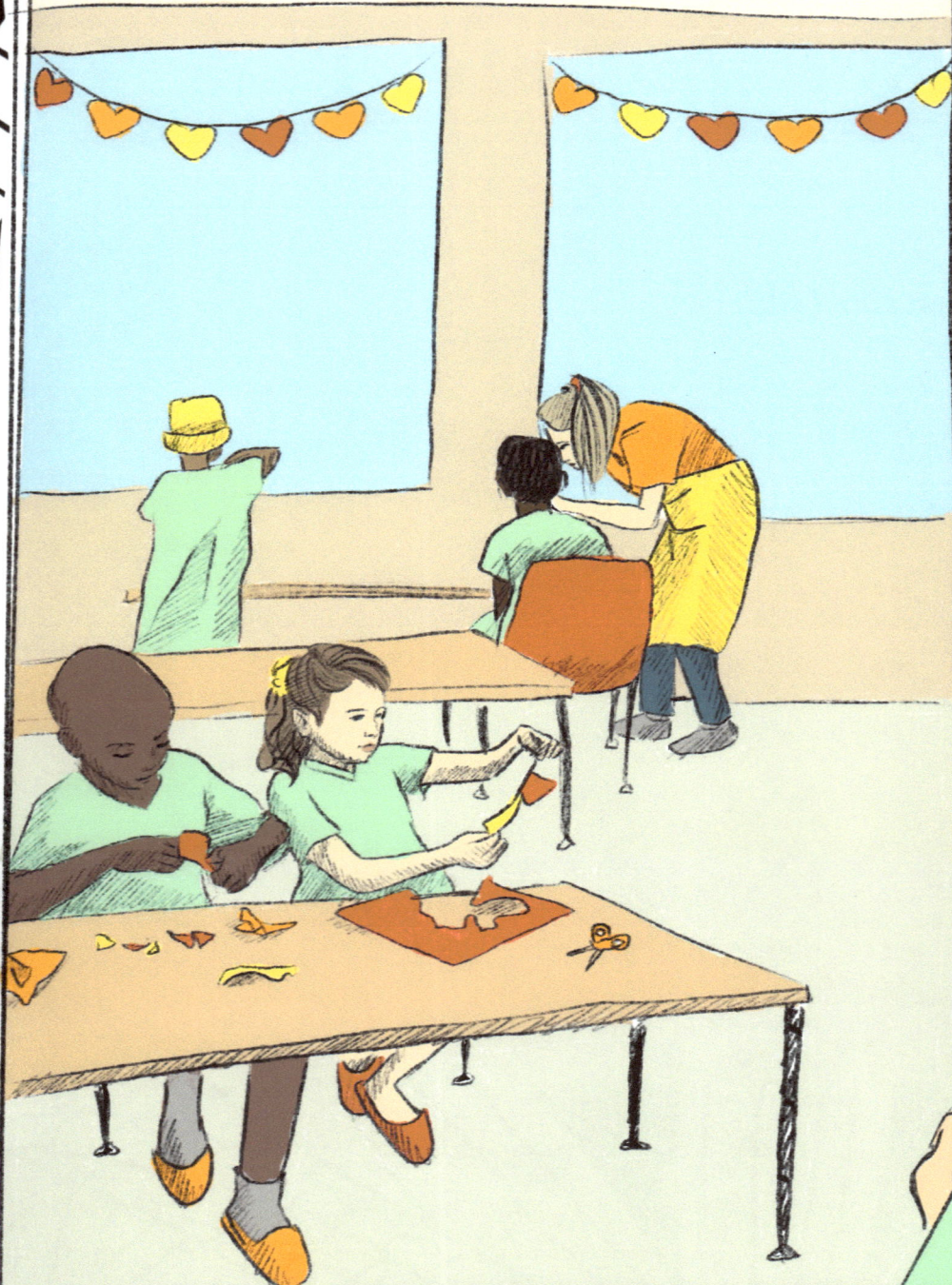

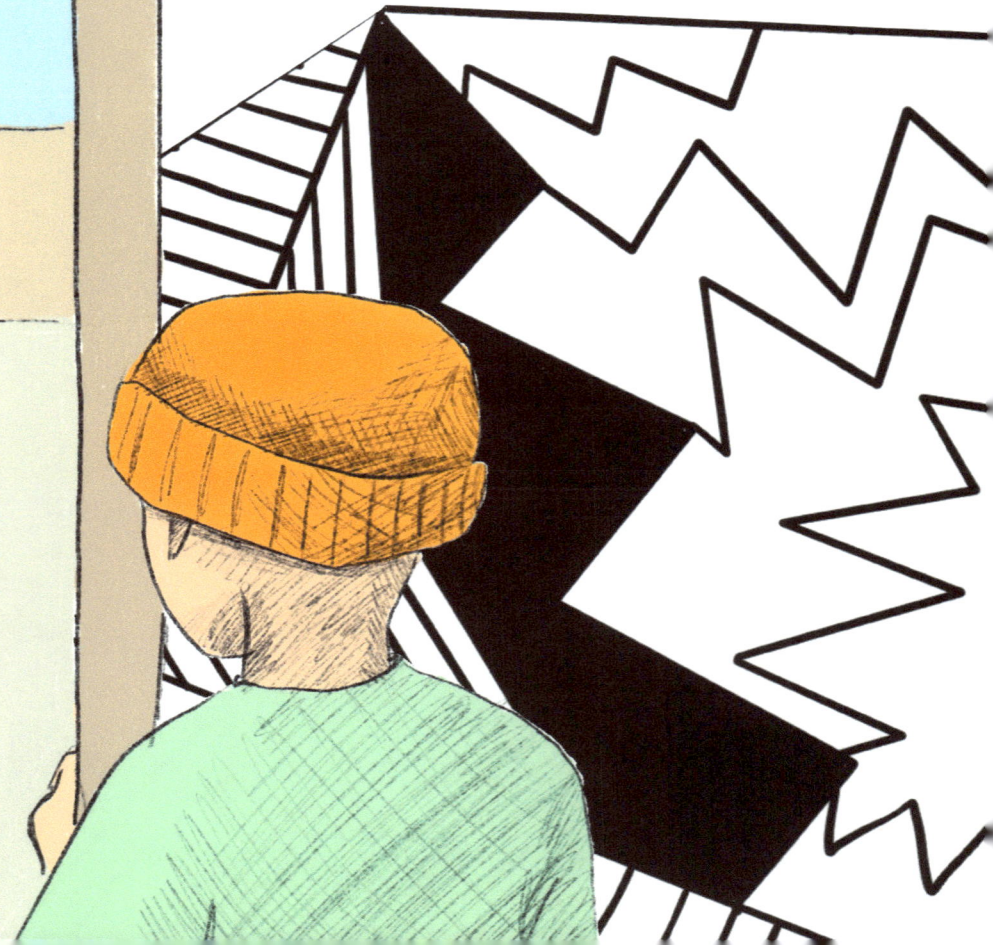

And to my surprise, I had a lot of fun! There were so many fun activities, and there was even a music room. Everyone was also very nice—they made me laugh and welcomed me to the clinic.

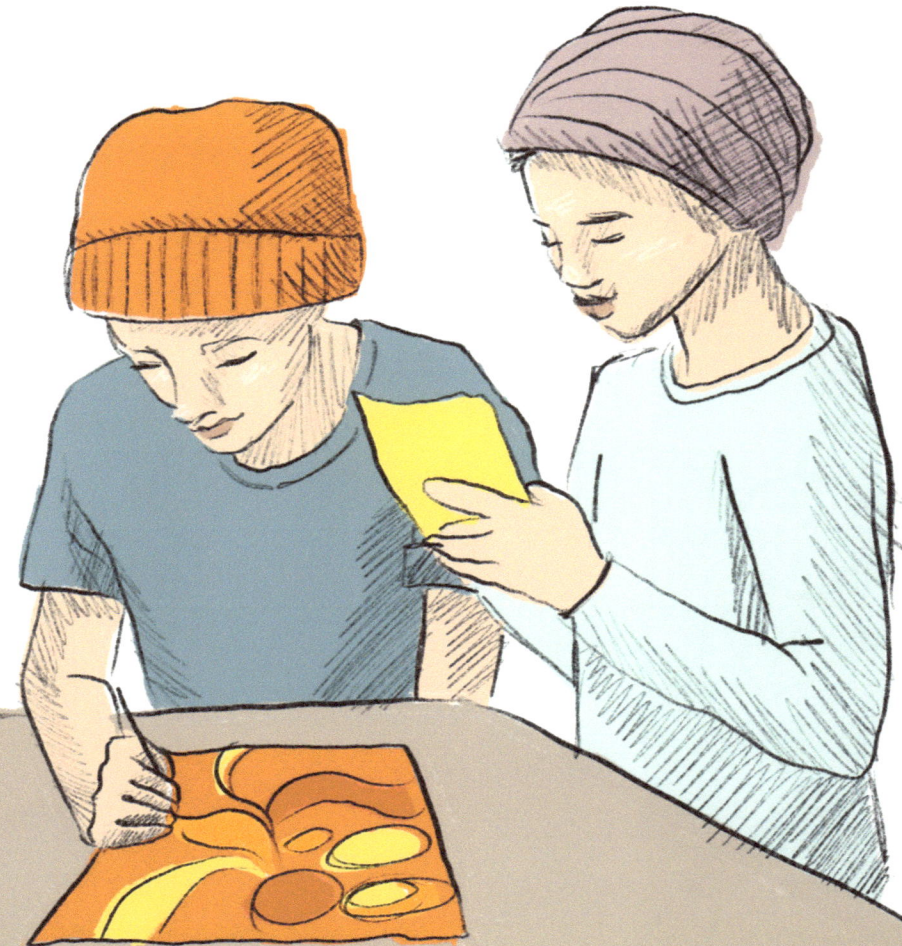

The first few rounds of chemotherapy went extremely well, especially with the encouragement of my friends in the activity room. I began to feel more confident about my treatment, except when they had to stick a needle inside of me. But it wasn't all bad; here's what happened:

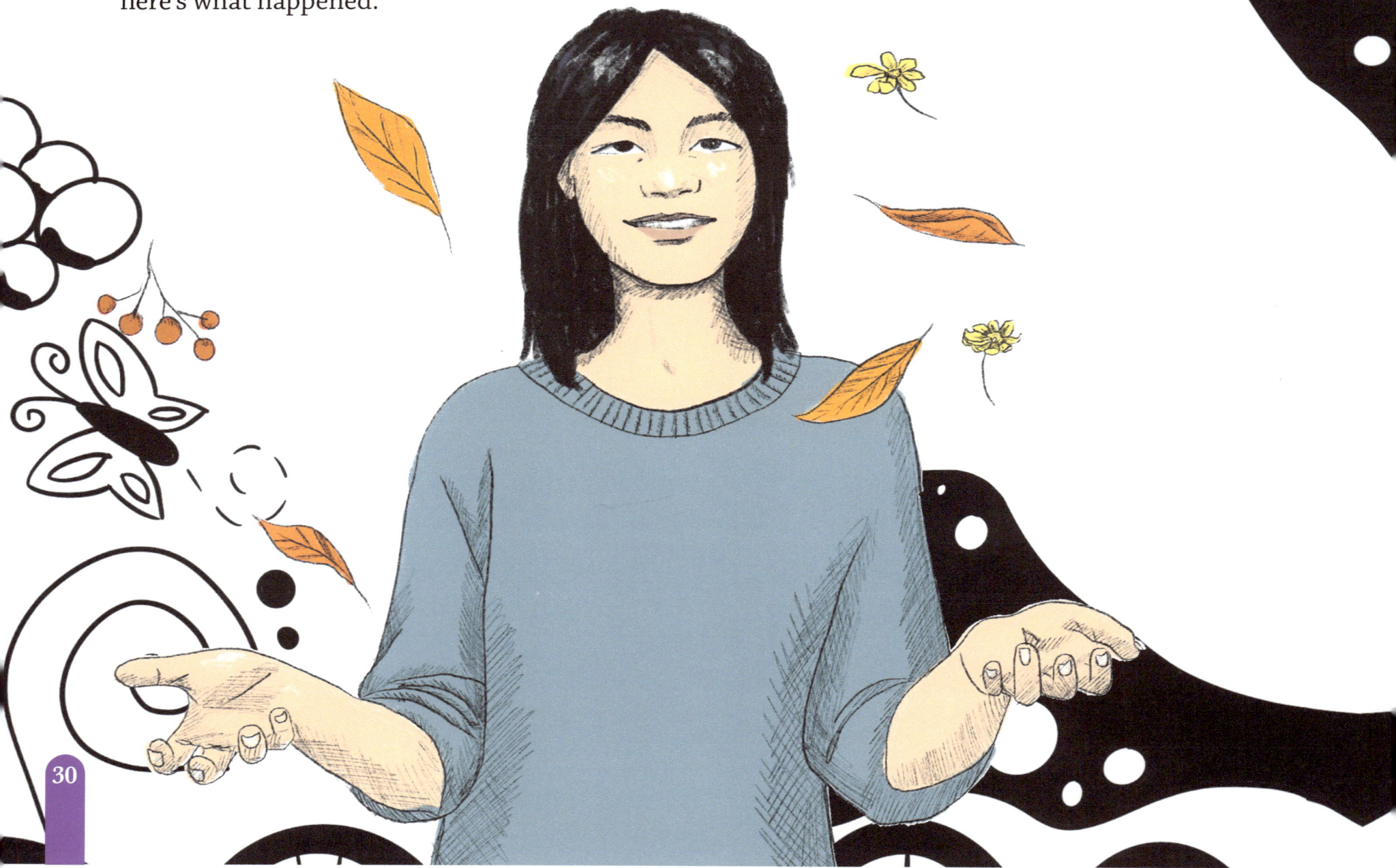

First, my mom applied a lidocaine cream that didn't make me feel anything.

Next, the nurses connected me to saline, a mixture of salt and water, to thin out the chemotherapy.

Finally, they hooked me up to chemotherapy!

Then, I sat there for a couple of hours as the medicine went inside me to do its job of making the cancer cells go away.

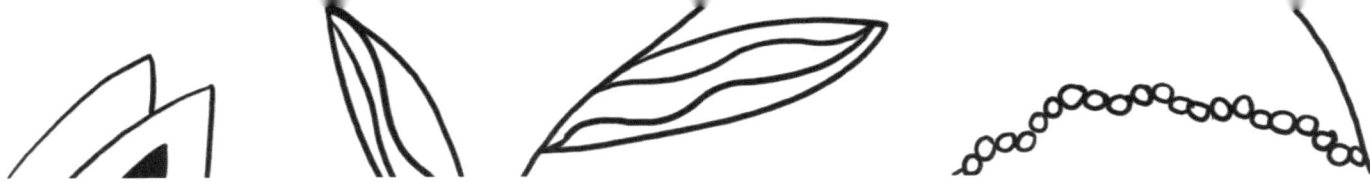

How did you feel after your first dose of chemotherapy?

_____

_____

Did you feel the same as you did before? Better? Worse?
Use this page to reflect on your experience.

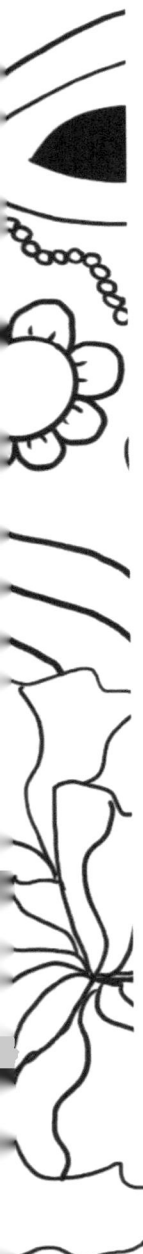

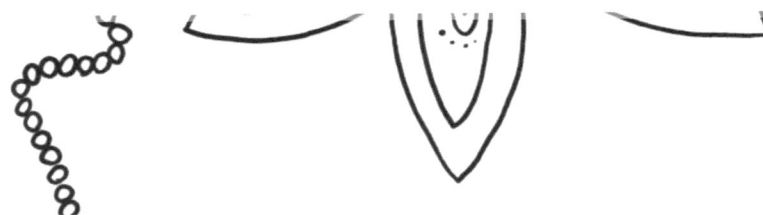

_____

_____

_____

_____

_____

_____

_____

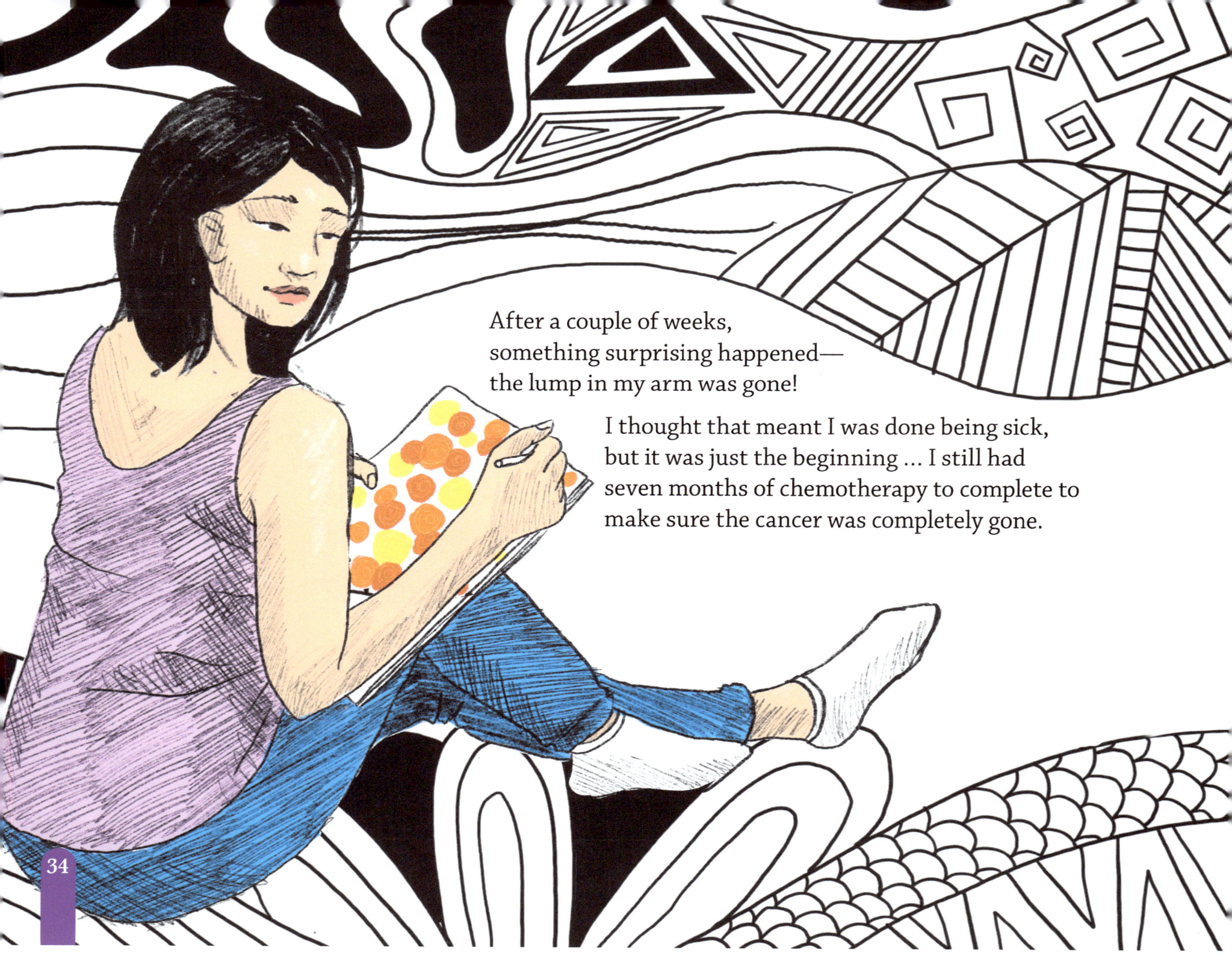

After a couple of weeks,
something surprising happened—
the lump in my arm was gone!

I thought that meant I was done being sick,
but it was just the beginning … I still had
seven months of chemotherapy to complete to
make sure the cancer was completely gone.

During the first month of chemotherapy, I shaved my head. I loved my hair, so I was embarrassed when I shaved it all off.

Here's what I looked like when I shaved my head.

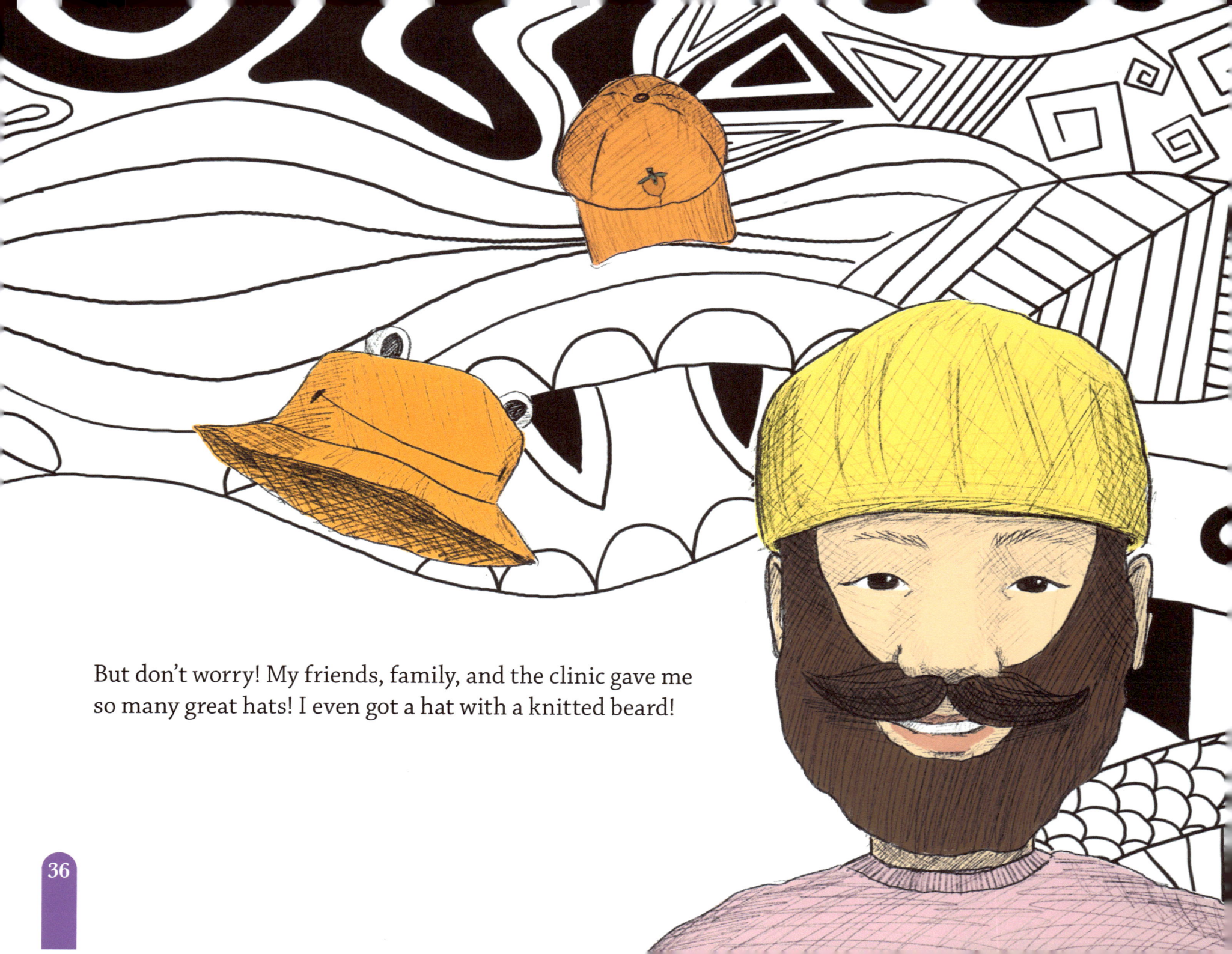

But don't worry! My friends, family, and the clinic gave me so many great hats! I even got a hat with a knitted beard!

Draw a picture of how you looked!

After a few weeks, I started experiencing the side effects of chemotherapy—I felt like throwing up all the time, and I was sore and in pain. But I was given extra medications to make me feel better.

During the first month of chemotherapy, some of my favorite moments were receiving cards and gifts full of good wishes. I felt so supported, and it made me happier.

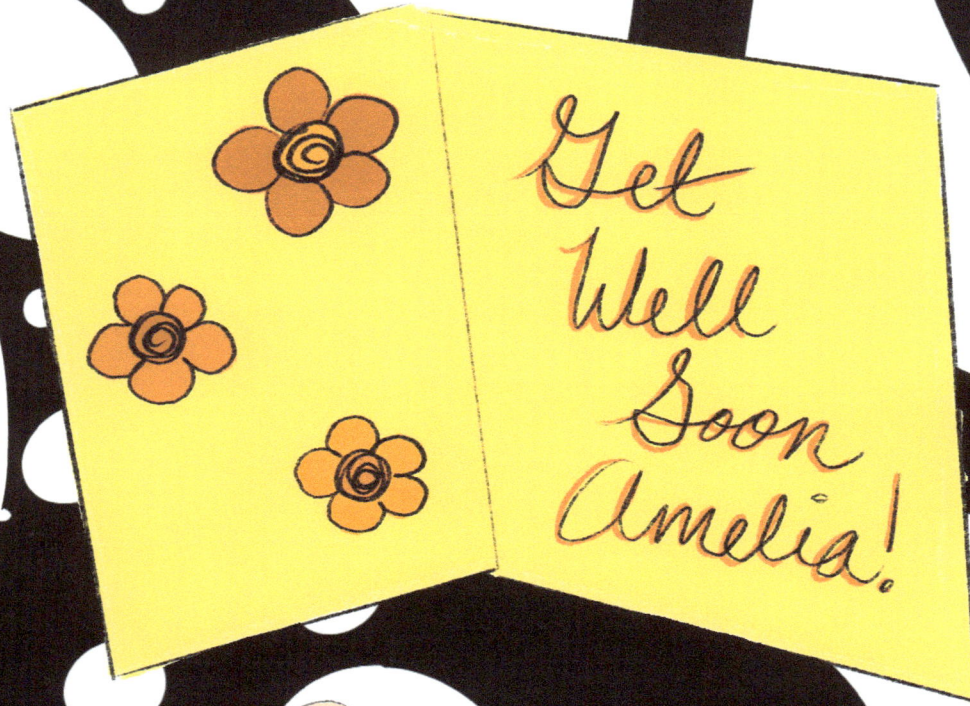

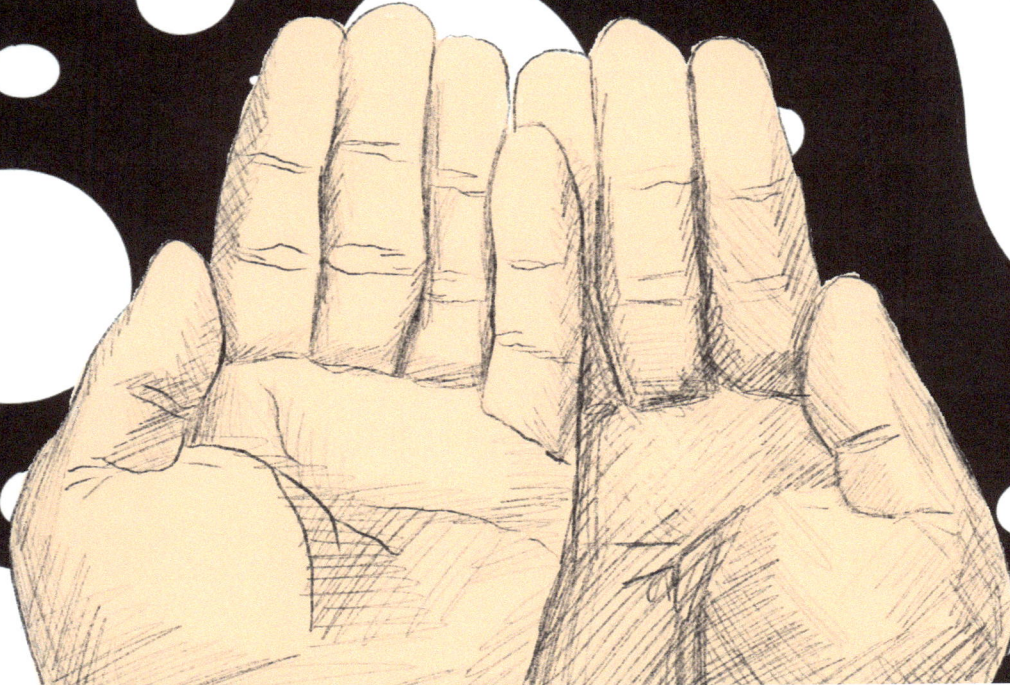

Get Well Soon Amelia!

One of my favorite memories, though, was when I met a new friend. She came all the way from China and was being treated for a brain tumor. I was sitting in the waiting room when my mom and her mother exchanged a few words. I got to know her, and we became friends. She introduced me to a fun game on my phone that warped our faces and made us laugh a lot.

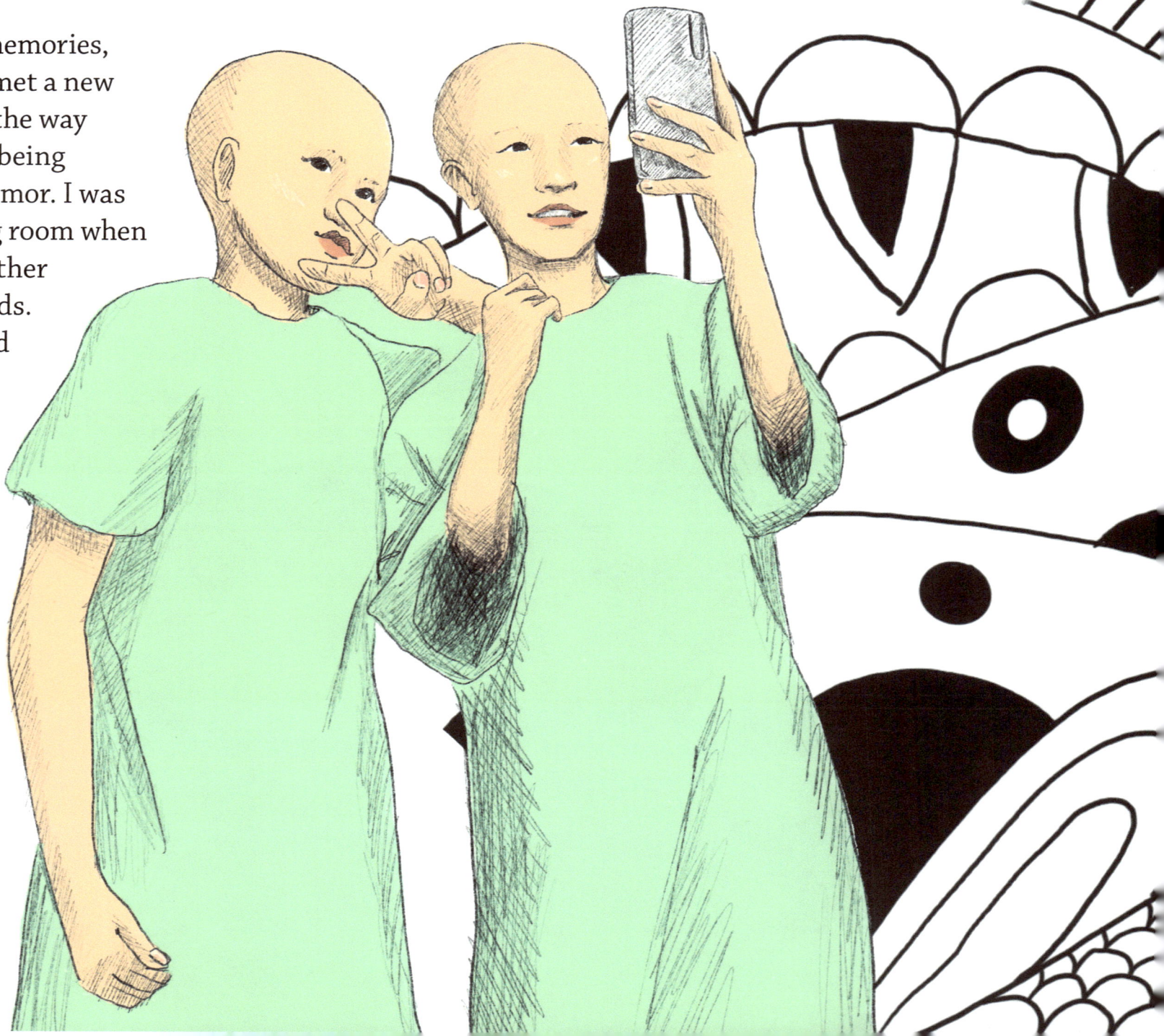

Have you met a special friend?

_____

_____

How did you meet them?

_____

_____

Why are they important to you?

_____

_____

_____

_____

_____

Having a friend was a very important part in my cancer journey. She understood what I was going through and told me that I was not alone.

The rest of chemotherapy was very similar to the end of the first month of chemo—I was still sick, but my view on life completely changed. Before chemotherapy, I never knew what it felt like to live in an unpredictable world. Now, I recognize that life is a gift that we should cherish and take advantage of. Would you like to color in my friends?

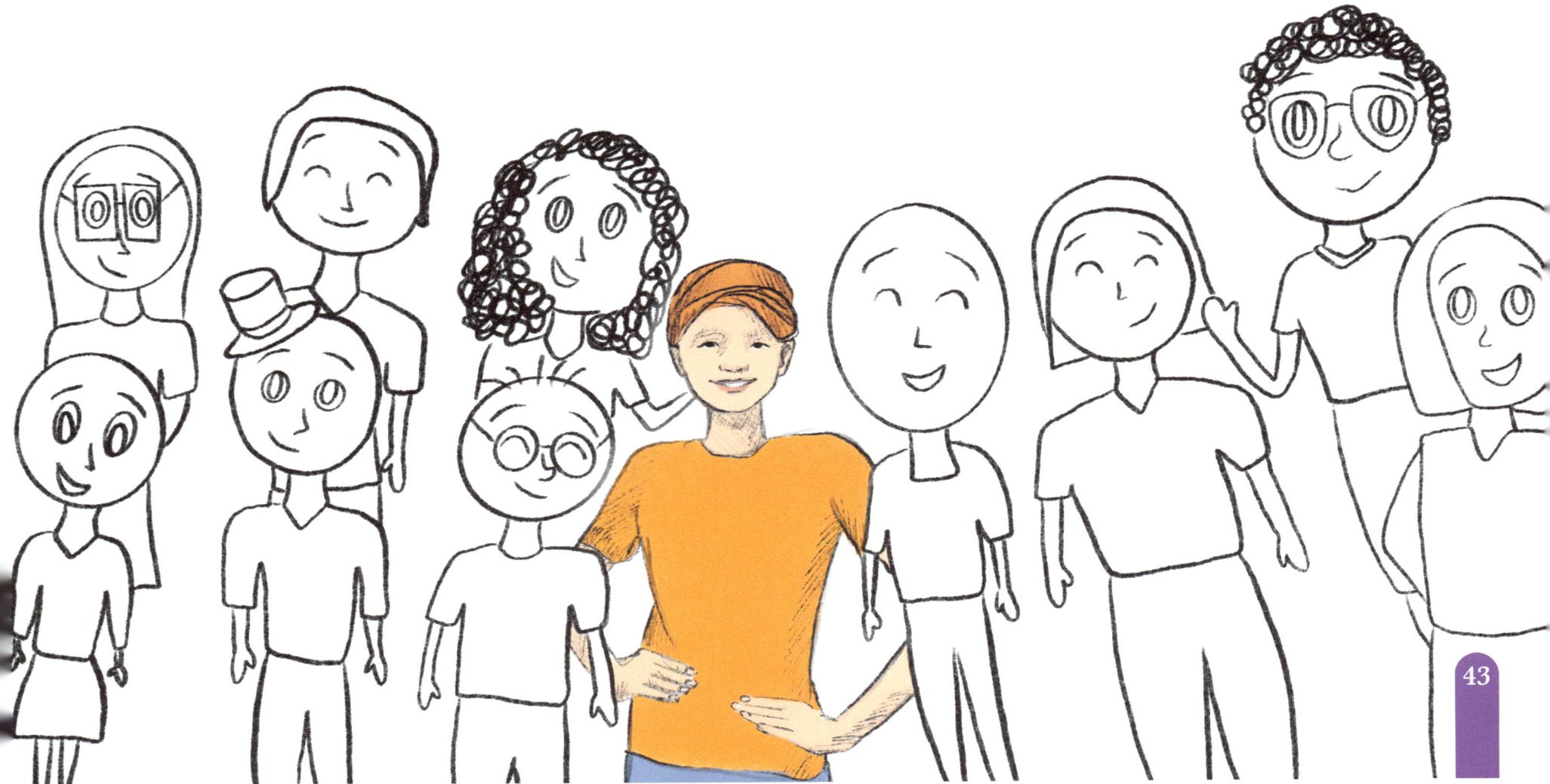

Here are a few things I learned …

1. *Try your best to approach everything in life with a positive mindset.*

2. *What it means to be loved.*
 ♺ *Who's sticking with you throughout your journey?*

3. *Being happy with yourself is true beauty.*

4. *You can tell people how you feel!*
 ♺ *Who is someone you can talk to when you're scared?*

5. *The support you receive from your friends and family is half the treatment.*
 ♺ Cancer can take away my hair and the color in my cheeks for a little while, but it can't take away the endless support my loved ones gave me.

Like how a thermometer checks your temperature, check on yourself and how you're feeling by asking yourself a few questions:

How are you feeling today?

_____

What is something you learned today?

_____

_____

What do you love about yourself?

_____

_____

What is something you found difficult today?

_____

_____

Acknowledgments

I would like to acknowledge my gratitude to Dr. Suzanne Forrest, Dr. Steven DuBois, and the rest of the staff at the Jimmy Fund Clinic. Their care, support, and zeal inspire me the most; I wouldn't be here today without them. I would also like to thank my friends and family for their constant support during and beyond my treatment.

I am forever grateful to Lisa Akoury-Ross, the publisher of SDP Publishing Solutions, LLC, Katie Barger, Olivia Bosson, Howard P. Johnson, and the rest of the publishing team. They are absolutely brilliant at what they do; this book is beyond what I imagined.

I am grateful to Taylor Russell, Dr. Stan Whitsett, Beth Raisner Glass, Hannah Arbuthnot, and the rest of the Make-A-Wish team for their funding and continued support. They have been there every step of the way and inspire me with their great work.

I'd like to give a special thanks to all my friends in the Jimmy Fund Clinic for showing me that I am strong and can do anything I put my mind to. For that, I am eternally grateful.

Finally, I want to thank my parents for all their help and long nights caring for me. I would not have made it through without their love and support.

About the Author

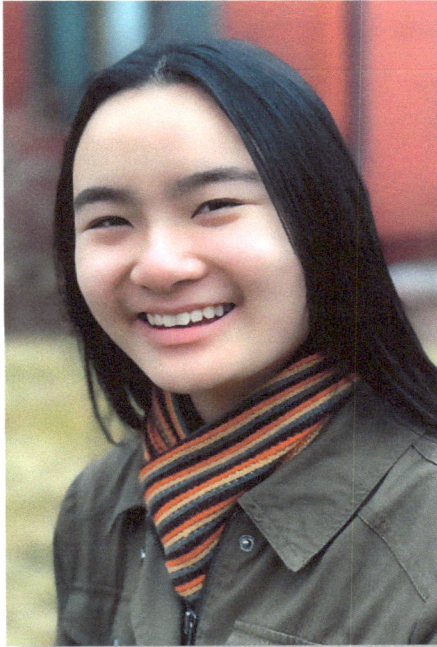

Amelia Zai is a former cancer patient at the Jimmy Fund Clinic in Boston, Massachusetts. Now, she is a rising college freshman who loves studying law, data science, and philosophy. Outside of school, she enjoys watching movies, cooking, and hanging out with her friends. Amelia chose to write this book as her wish through Make-A-Wish®, to remind all young cancer patients that they are not alone and that the journey is more important than the final destination. Further, she wants this interactive journal to be a token of her gratitude to all who supported her during her cancer journey.

All author proceeds will be donated to Make-A-Wish® Massachusetts and Rhode Island to support its mission of creating life-changing wishes for children with critical illnesses.

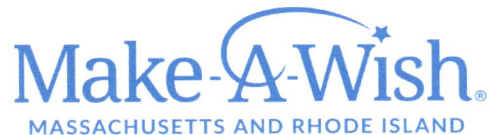

Make-A-Wish.®
MASSACHUSETTS AND RHODE ISLAND

www.massri.wish.org

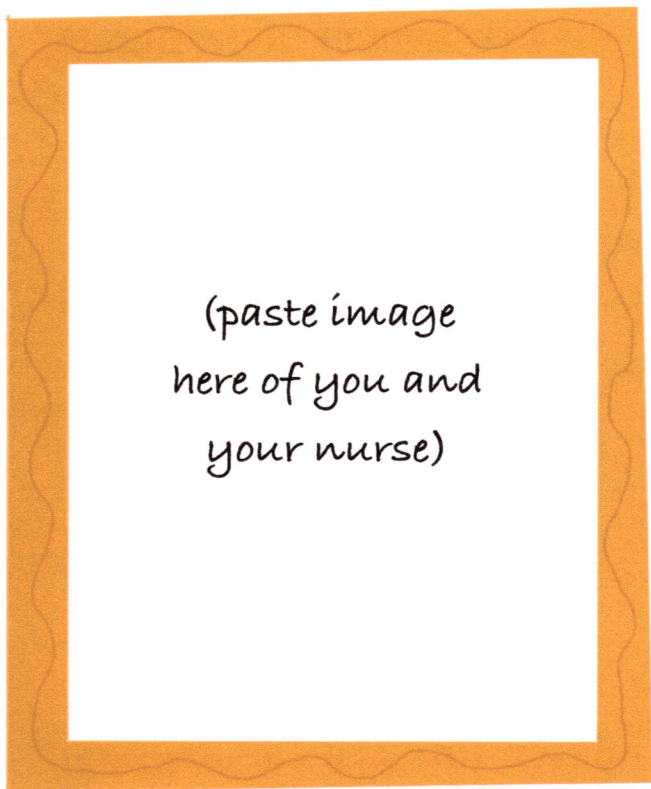

(paste image here of you and
your nurse)

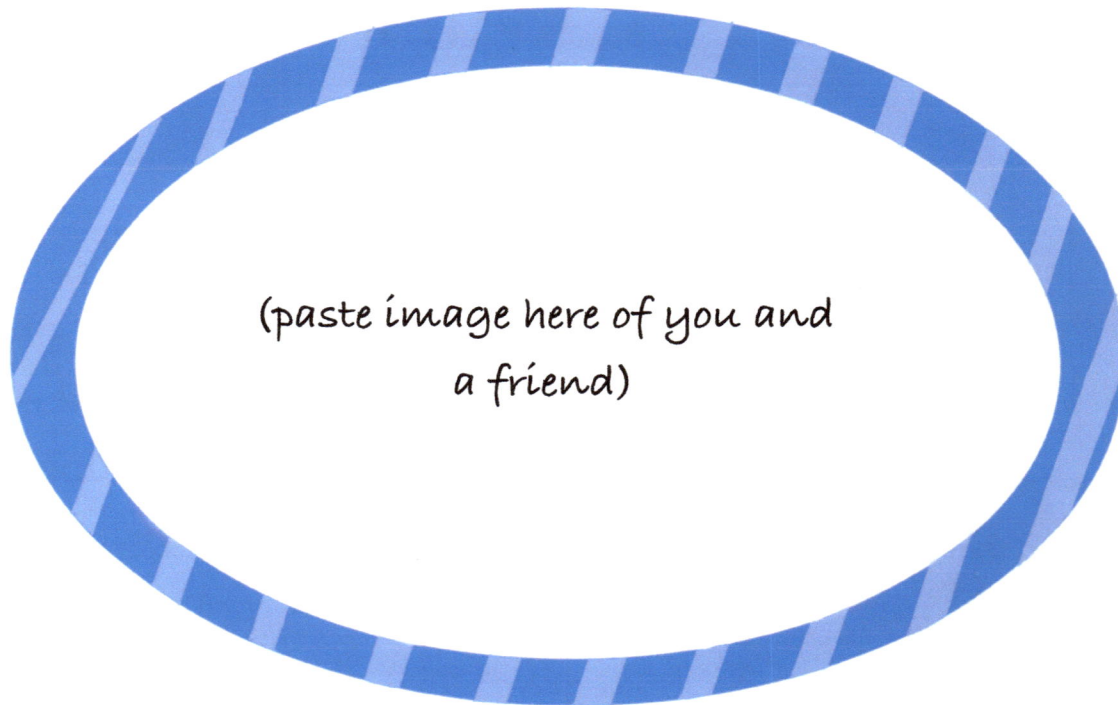

(paste image here of you and
a friend)

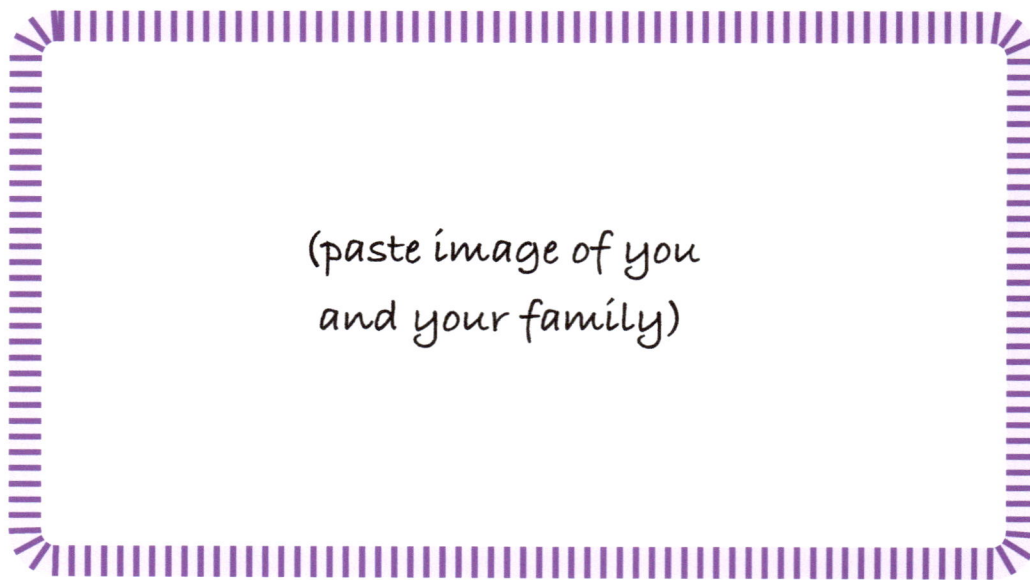

(paste image of you
and your family)

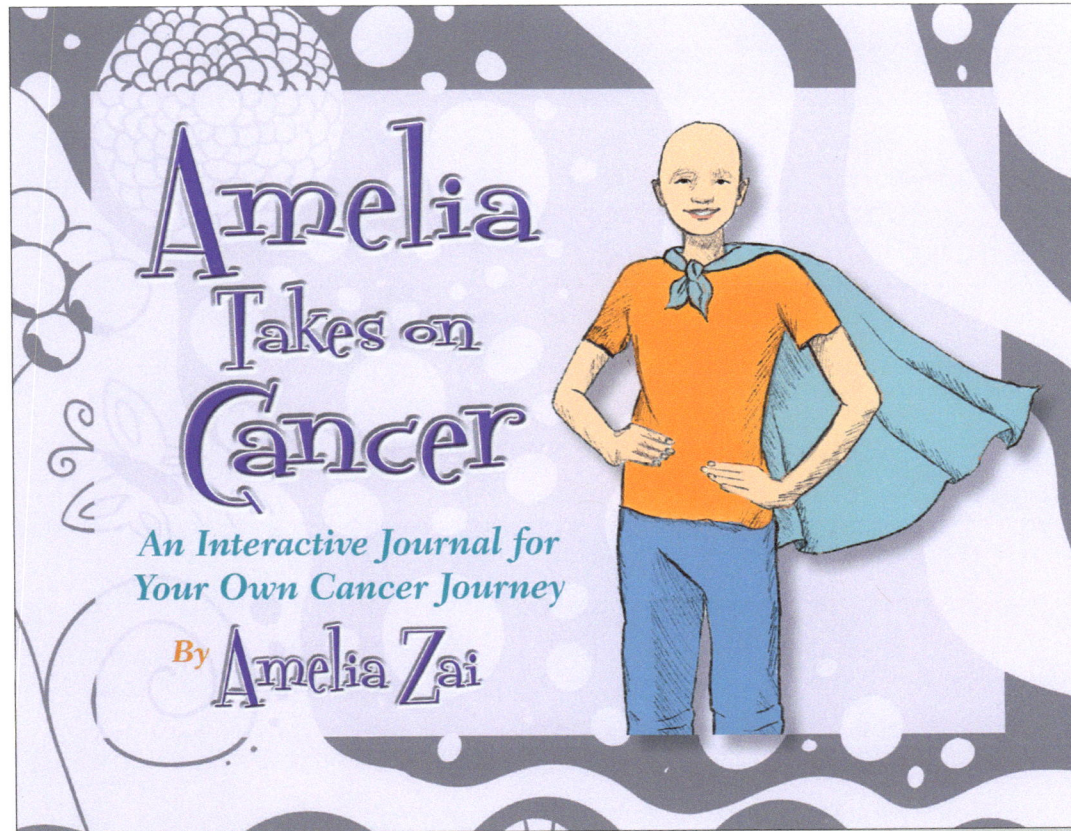

Amelia Takes on Cancer
An Interactive Journal for Your Own Cancer Journey
Amelia Zai

Publisher: SDP Publishing
Also available in ebook format
Available at all major bookstores

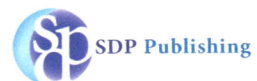
SDP Publishing

www.SDPPublishing.com
Contact us at: info@SDPPublishing.com

www.ingramcontent.com/pod-product-compliance
Lightning Source LLC
Chambersburg PA
CBHW041651260326

41914CB00017B/1612